Essential Mediterranean Sea Recipes Selection

Delicious & Creative Mediterranean Meals

Mateo Buscema

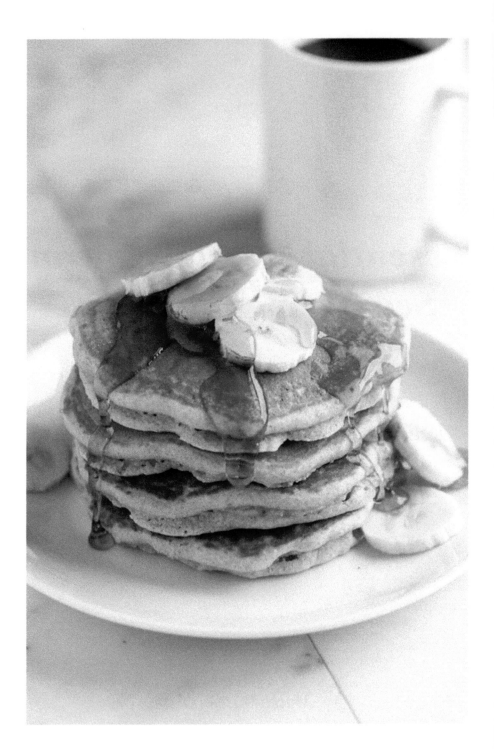

TABLE OF CONTENTS

Tex-Mex omelet with roasted cherry tomato salsa

omelet is fully stuffed with black beans, chips topped with roasted cherry tomato salsa. It is perfect for breakfast, dinner and lunch in only 40 minutes.

Ingredients

- ⅓ cup of loosely packed cilantro, chopped
- 2 cloves garlic, minced
- 1 small lime, juiced
- Sliced avocado
- ⅛ teaspoon of sea salt
- 2 tablespoons of milk or water
- Hot sauce
- Pinch of sea salt
- Pinch of black pepper
- Sour cream
- Hot sauce
- 1 pint of cherry tomatoes
- 1 jalapeño, deseeded and membranes removed chopped
- 1 scant tablespoon butter
- ⅓ cup Jack cheese or other melty cheese

- ½ small white onion, chopped
- 3 tablespoons black beans
- 2 eggs
- ½ teaspoon of olive oil
- handful blue corn chips or tortilla chips, broken into small pieces

Directions

1. start by making the salsa by preheating the oven to 400°F.
2. Line a small, rimmed baking pan with parchment paper for easy cleaning.
3. Toss the cherry tomatoes and ½ teaspoon of olive oil together with a Sprinkle of sea salt on the baking pan.
4. Roast for 15 – 20 minutes to the extent the tomatoes are juicy and collapsing easily.
5. In another separate bowl, mix together the cilantro, chopped onion, jalapeño, lime juice or vinegar, garlic, and sea salt.
6. Use a serrated knife to chop the tomatoes once they have cooled off.
7. Pull off the tomato skins for a smoother salsa.
8. Mix the tomatoes into the mixture.
9. Taste and season accordingly.
10. Secondly, it is time to make the omelet.
11. In a bowl, whisk together the milk or water, eggs, black pepper, sea salt, and dashes of hot sauce.

12. Heat a well-seasoned cast iron skillet over medium-low heat.

13. Add a drop of water sizzles on contact when the skillet is hot.

14. Toss in the pat of butter tilt to all sides to coat.

15. Pour in the egg mixture and let it set for briefly.

16. Using a spatula, scoot the eggs toward the middle of the pan, make sure to tilt the pan so runny eggs take their place.

17. Repeat this process until there is hardly any runny eggs to scoot.

18. Using your spatula again, release the underside of the omelet from the pan.

19. Keep tilting the pan to prevent the omelet form sticking on the pan.

20. Let it set briefly, then scoop it off the pan to a plate

21. Immediately top ½ of the warm omelet with a sprinkle of cheese.

22. Then with smashed tortilla chips, black beans, and more cheese.

23. Gently fold the other half on top.

24. Spoon a generous amount of salsa over the middle of the omelet.

25. Serve immediately and enjoy.

Banana trail mix

Coconut, oats, naturally sweetened honey give this recipe an elevated taste. Feel free to top this banana trail mix bread with nuts, dry fruits and serve with Greek yogurt to pull out all the sweetness to excite your taste buds.

Ingredients

- ¼ cup of honey
- 1 large egg
- ¾ cup of whole wheat pastry flour
- ¼ cup of chopped dark chocolate
- ½ cup of oats
- 1 ½ teaspoons of baking powder
- ½ cup of virgin coconut oil, melted
- 1 tablespoon of turbinado sugar
- 1 teaspoon of vanilla extract
- ½ cup of pecans, toasted and chopped
- ½ teaspoon of cinnamon
- ¾ cup of unsweetened shredded coconut, divided
- ⅓ cup of chopped candied ginger
- ⅓ cup of chopped dried cherries or cranberries
- ¼ teaspoon of table salt

- 1 cup of mashed ripe banana

Directions

1. Expressly begin by preheating your oven to 375°F.
2. Grease your loaf pan.
3. In a medium sized bowl, whisk the flour together with, baking powder, oats, salt and cinnamon.
4. Stir in ½ cup of shredded coconut, immediately mix in the pecans, chopped ginger, dried fruit, and dark chocolate.
5. In a separate bowl, also whisk the coconut oil together with the mashed banana, egg, honey, and vanilla.
6. Mix the wet ingredients together with the dry ingredients keep stirring until properly combined.
7. Place the batter into the loaf pan.
8. Sprinkle with the remaining ¼ cup of coconut.
9. Then top with a light sprinkle of turbinado (raw) sugar.
10. Bake until the toothpick inserted into the center comes out clean in 50 minutes.
11. Allow the bread cool in the pan, then you can slice.
12. Serve and enjoy.

Maple cinnamon applesauce

An apple a say keeps the doctor far away!!! In 20 minutes you will be able to keep the doctor as far away as possible. Serve it with oat meal or pancakes for a nutritious healthy breakfast.

Ingredients

- 1 tablespoon of ground cinnamon
- ¼ cup of and 2 tablespoons real maple syrup
- Dash of sea salt
- 3 Gala apples
- 1 tablespoon of fresh lemon juice
- 3 Granny Smith or pippin apples

Directions

1. Of course you must start by peeling, core and chopping the apples into chunks.
2. In a heavy Dutch oven heated to a medium temperature, combine the apple chunks, together with the cinnamon, maple syrup, and lemon juice.
3. Cover tightly and let simmer for 12 minutes to soften the apples slightly.

4. Uncover the pot, continue cooking as you stir occasionally to break up the larger chunks in 5 – 10 minutes or accordingly.
5. Remove from heat source, you can add more maple syrup, cinnamon or lemon juice to suit your taste.
6. Serve warm or chilled.
7. Enjoy.
8. Keep leftover in the fridge after is has cooled to room temperature.

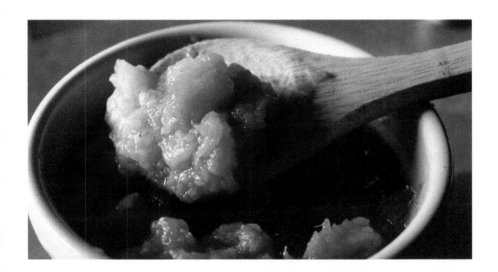

Baked asparagus frittata

This is one of a kind beautiful baked asparagus frittata recipe, very easy to make yet can make 6 larger servings.

Ingredients

- Pinch of sea salt
- 1 ½ teaspoons of Dijon mustard
- ⅓ cup of milk
- ½ cup of crumbled goat cheese
- 6 large eggs
- Handful of thin asparagus
- Drizzle olive oil
- Big pinch salt
- Heaping tablespoon finely chopped shallot
- Big squeeze fresh lemon juice
- Freshly ground black pepper

Directions

1. Preheat oven to 400°F.
2. Secondly, line a baking pan with two strips of parchment paper trimmed to fit.

3. In a medium sized bowl, scramble the eggs together with the shallot, milk, mustard, goat cheese, and salt.
4. Pour the egg mixture into the prepared baking pan.
5. Carefully slide it onto the middle rack of the oven.
6. Bake for 10 minutes.
7. As the eggs are baking, rinse the asparagus and pat dry.
8. Trim off the tough ends of the asparagus.
9. Toss the asparagus with a big squeeze of lemon juice, salt, a drizzle of olive oil, and pepper.
10. Keep aside for later.
11. In 10 minutes, remove the egg dish from the oven.
12. Place the asparagus, one by one, on top.
13. Return back the rack to the oven for 15 minutes.
14. Let the frittata rest for a few minutes.
15. Next, slide a knife around the edges of the pan
16. Using both your hands, lift the frittata out and put onto a flat surface.
17. With a sharp knife slice it in three columns, in between the strips of asparagus.
18. Gently slice down the middle, through the asparagus.
19. Serve warm or at room temperature.
20. Enjoy.

Buckwheat and spelt crepes

Using a food processor these crepes are easier to whip, or even by hand and they really do not take long to get ready. They are blessed with a nutty flavor and amazing with savory eggs, butter and some fruity fillings. In 22 minutes your buckwheat and spelt crepes will be ready for breakfast, dinner and or desert depending on how you like it.

Ingredients

- ¾ cup of plus 2 tablespoons milk
- 1 tablespoon of unsalted butter, melted
- ¼ cup of buckwheat flour
- ½ cup of whole spelt flour
- 2 large eggs
- ¼ teaspoon of salt
- 2 teaspoons of sugar

Directions

1. In a food processor, combine the sugar, flours, and salt.
2. Pulse it briefly to combine.
3. Add the milk to the content together with the eggs and melted butter.

4. Pour the liquid ingredients into the food processor blend till the mixture is uniform.

5. Keeping scraping down the sides during the mixing procedure.

6. Heat a medium-sized pan over medium temperature.

7. When the pan is hot enough, pour in some of the melted butter.

8. Spread the butter evenly.

9. Use a ¼ cup measuring cup to ladle batter into the pan.

10. Swirl the batter around the pan to ensure it is equally distributed through the surface.

11. Cook the crepe until the bottom is firm and speckled with brown spots within 1 minute.

12. Now, loosen the edges and flip the crepe to cook the other side in the same time (1 minute).

13. Put on a plate when the crepe is speckled and golden on both sides.

14. Keep repeating this step until all the batter is used up.

15. When you are done, serve and enjoy.

Cranberry orange steel cut oats

Oats as nutritious as they are, they form a whole grain meal for breakfast served with yogurt, you will love and aroma and taste.

Ingredients

- Juice of one orange
- Toasted and chopped pecans or yogurt
- 3 cups of water
- 1 cup of almond milk
- 1 cup of steel-cut oats
- Zest of one orange
- ¼ teaspoon of salt
- 1 tablespoon of unsalted butter
- Cranberry sauce

Directions

1. In a large saucepan, bring the water to boil together with the milk over a medium simmering temperature.
2. As the mixture boils, melt the butter in a skillet over medium heat.
3. Toast the oats while stirring occasionally to obtain a golden and fragrant within 2 minutes.

4. Stir the oats gently into the simmering water and milk mixture.
5. Lower the heat to medium low let it simmer for 20 minutes till when thick.
6. Stir in the salt.
7. Continue to simmer the mixture to absorb all the liquid in 10 minutes.
8. Stir in the orange zest and juice, let the oatmeal settle for 5 minutes.
9. Portion into dishes and top with cranberry sauce and then ensure to toast with a splash of almond milk, pecans, or Greek yogurt.
10. Serve and enjoy.

Baked oatmeal with blackberries, coconut and bananas

Packed with several fruits, this baked oatmeal is a perfect Mediterranean Sea diet healthy for anyone. You are also at liberty to serve with any berry of your liking. Your meal will take up to 1 hour but trust me it is worth holding up for that much time.

Ingredients

- ½ cup of unsweetened shredded coconut
- 2 ripe bananas, cut into ½-inch pieces
- 1 big egg
- 1 ½ cups of blackberries
- Scant ½ teaspoon of fine-grain sea salt
- 1 can of light coconut milk
- ⅓ cup of pure maple syrup (or raw sugar)
- 1 ½ teaspoons of ground cinnamon
- 2 cups of rolled oats
- 3 tablespoons of unsalted butter, melted
- 2 teaspoons of pure vanilla extract

- 1 teaspoon of aluminum-free baking powder
- ⅓ cup of water

Directions

1. Preheat your oven to 375°F.
2. Put a rack in the top third of the oven.
3. Spray cooking oil on the inside of the baking dish.
4. In a medium sized bowl, mix together the coconut, cinnamon, oats, sugar, baking powder, and salt.
5. In a separate bowl, whisk the maple syrup together with the half of the butter, coconut milk, egg, water, and the vanilla.
6. Place the banana slices in a single layer on the bottom of the baking dish.
7. Organize 2/3 of the berries on top of the bananas.
8. Cover the fruit with the dry oat mixture.
9. Drizzle the wet ingredients over the oats.
10. Shake the baking dish to allow the milk move down through the oats.
11. Scatter the remaining berries across the top.
12. Sprinkle some extra coconut flakes and raw sugar on top (optional)
13. Start baking for 45 minutes make the top is golden.
14. Remove the baked oatmeal off heat source.
15. Set aside to let cool for briefly.
16. Drizzle the remaining melted butter on the top.

17. Serve and enjoy.

Basic baked frittata recipe

Ingredients

- A handful of cheese
- A splash of milk
- Spices
- 6 eggs
- Salt
- Vegetables
- Pepper

Directions

1. Get your oven preheated to 400°F.
2. Line your pan which must be spring form pan with parchment paper.
3. In a separate bowl or dish, whisk eggs together with the milk, cheese, vegetables and all the seasonings.
4. Pour the mixture into the spring form pan.
5. Bake until the frittata is golden and puffy.
6. The center should feel firm and springy within 25 minutes.
7. Serve and enjoy.

Southwestern corn chowder

Over a stovetop in 50 or 0 minutes this corn chowder will be ready for serving for a cozy dinner. This recipe is entirely vegetarian and wholesomely finger licking delicious.

Ingredients

- 1 large red onion, chopped
- 1 poblano pepper seeds and ribs removed and chopped
- 1 red bell pepper, chopped
- ¼ cup of crème fraiche or sour cream
- Freshly ground black pepper
- 2 tablespoons of unsalted butter, cut into 4 pieces
- 2 celery ribs, chopped
- 1 tablespoon of extra-virgin olive oil
- ¾ teaspoon of salt, divided
- 1 tablespoon of fresh lime juice
- ½ teaspoon of chili powder
- ¼ cup of chopped cilantro
- 2 medium cloves garlic, pressed
- 4 cups of vegetable broth
- 1 pound of red potatoes, cut into ¾" cubes
- 2 cups of water

- 1 bay leaf
- ears of fresh sweet corn, shucked

Directions

1. In a medium soup pot, warm the olive oil over medium temperature to the point of shimmering without smoke.
2. Add the onion, potatoes, corn, poblano, celery, bell pepper, ½ teaspoon of salt, and ½ teaspoon chili powder.
3. Stir to enable it combine well.
4. Cook until the onions are tender and translucent in 7 – 10 minutes while stirring occasionally.
5. Introduce in the garlic and cook until fragrant in 1 minute, while stirring constantly.
6. Add the broth and water, stir to combine.
7. Place in the bay leaf.
8. Bring to a boil over high heat.
9. Reduce the heat after some time to allow simmering for 20 – 25 minutes, stirring occasionally until the potatoes are easily pierced
10. Remove the pot from the heat source.
11. Carefully remove the bay leaf using a kitchen tong.
12. Carefully transfer 3 cups of the soup to a blender.
13. Fasten the lid tight enough not to let steam escape, then blend until completely smooth.
14. Add the butter and blend again.

15. Pour the mixture back into the pot.
16. Add the crème fraiche, cilantro, and lime juice stir to combine.
17. Next, season with the remaining ¼ teaspoon of salt and black pepper, taste and continue to season accordingly.
18. Separate the chowder into bowls and top with garnishes of your choice.
19. Serve and enjoy.
20. The left over can be kept in a refrigerator for up to 5 days.

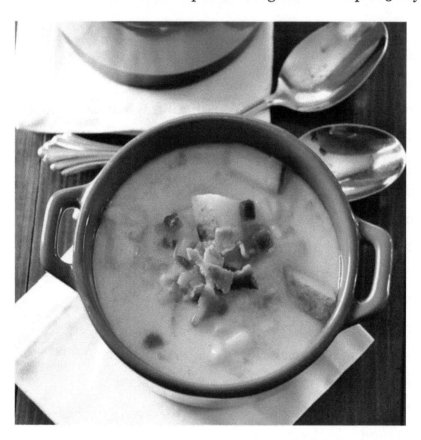

Veggie sesame noodles

Several colorful vegetables form a remarkable part of this recipe. As a result, it is known to be healthy and easy to prepare in 35 minutes. It is gluten-free Mediterranean Sea diet that can yield 6 side servings.

Ingredients

- 1 bunch of green onions, chopped
- ½ cup of chopped cilantro
- ½ teaspoon of red pepper flakes
- ¼ cup of raw sesame seeds
- ¼ cup of toasted sesame oil
- 2 cups of shelled edamame, steamed
- 1 teaspoon of grated fresh ginger
- 2 ½ cups of thinly sliced red cabbage
- 3 whole carrots, peeled and then sliced into ribbons
- 1 red bell pepper, sliced strips
- 2 cloves garlic, pressed
- ⅓ cup of reduced sodium tamari
- 2 tablespoons of lime juice
- ounces of soba noodles

Directions

1. Cook the soba noodles as instructed on the package.
2. Drain out any excess water in a colander and rinse them well with cool water.
3. Move the drained noodles to a large serving bowl, keep aside for later.
4. Toast the sesame seeds in a small skillet over medium temperature keep stirring frequently.
5. When they are fragrant and turned golden move them to a small bowl and also keep aside for later.
6. In another separate bowl, combine the tamari, lime juice, sesame oil, garlic, ginger, and red pepper flakes blend together at once until fully blended keep aside for later.
7. Add the carrots, cabbage, green onions, bell pepper, cilantro and optional edamame to assemble with the noodles in a bowl.
8. Drizzle in the dressing.
9. Add all of the sesame seeds, and use tongs to toss until the mixture is fully combined.
10. Serve immediately and enjoy.
11. Any leftovers can be kept in the refrigerator for later.

Pasta alla Norma

This pasta is Sicilian but so delicious that you may not resist it. It is combined with eggplants, basil and marinara. The eggplants are specifically roasted to suite the recipe and bring out the best taste.

Ingredients

- ½ teaspoon dried oregano
- ¼ cup plus 1 teaspoon extra-virgin olive oil
- ½ cup chopped fresh basil, plus a handful basil leaves
- ¼ teaspoon fine salt, more to taste
- 2 medium eggplants
- ½ to 1 teaspoon red pepper flakes
- ounces of rigatoni, ziti or spaghetti
- 1 batch Super Simple Marinara Sauce
- ¾ cup of finely grated ricotta salata

Directions

1. Cook the marinara sauce as instructed on the package.
2. When the marinara is ready, cover the pot and keep it warm over very low heat.
3. As the marinara is getting ready, preheat your oven to 425°F. make sure there are racks in the upper and lower thirds of the oven.
4. Line two large, rimmed baking sheets with parchment paper for easy cleanup.
5. Shave off long alternating strips of eggplant peel with a vegetable peeller.
6. Then slice the eggplants into ½-inch thick rounds throw the unwanted pieces.

7. Place the eggplant on the lined baking sheets.
8. Brush the with olive oil on every side.
9. Sprinkle the with salt and lots of pepper.
10. Roast until deeply golden and tender in 40 – 45 minutes, flip after 20 minutes to roast the other side.
11. Boil a large pot of salted water, place in the pasta let cook till al dente as directed on the package. Reserve some pasta cooking water.
12. Return the pasta to the pot after draining.
13. Gently stir the roasted eggplant into the sauce.
14. Add the remaining 1 teaspoon olive oil, red pepper flakes, fresh basil.
15. Crush the dried oregano between your fingers add to the content.
16. Add the pasta to the sauce with a couple tablespoons of the reserved pasta water, stir.
17. Add 2/3 of the cheese.
18. Season to taste with salt and black pepper.
19. Divide the pasta in 4 bowls.
20. Sprinkle cheese on top of the individual servings and some extra fresh basil.
21. Serve and enjoy.

Quick Chana masala

Quick Chana masala is best served over rice preferably basmati rice. Much as its genesis can be traced back to India, it is a gluten free vegan recipe and a perfect Mediterranean Sea diet. Endeavor to prepare the ingredients prior to preparing the recipe.

Ingredients

- 1 ½ teaspoons of garam masala
- 1 medium yellow onion, chopped
- 1 tablespoon of peeled and minced ginger
- ½ teaspoon of sea salt
- 5 cloves garlic, pressed
- 1 large can fire-roasted crushed tomatoes
- 1 ½ teaspoons of ground coriander
- ¾ teaspoon of ground cumin
- 2 tablespoons of coconut oil or extra-virgin olive oil
- 1 cup of uncooked brown basmati rice
- Fresh cilantro
- 1 medium serrano or jalapeño pepper
- Pinch of cayenne pepper
- 2 cans of chickpeas

- ½ teaspoon of ground turmeric
- Lemon wedges

Directions

1. Start by cooking the rice for serving the Chana masala
2. Bring a large pot of water to boil, add the rice after the begins to boil
3. Boil the rice for 30 minutes put off the heat and drain the rice.
4. Return the rice to the pot and cover the pot, let simmer for 10 minutes.
5. Remove the lid, fluff the rice with a fork and season with sea salt accordingly.
6. Next, cook the Chana masala
7. In a large size saucepan, warm the oil over medium-low heat.
8. Add the serrano, onion, and salt.
9. Cook until the onion turns translucent within 5 minutes.
10. Add the garlic together with the ginger.
11. Continue to cook for 1 minute until fragrant.
12. Stir in the garam masala, cumin, turmeric, coriander, salt and cayenne.
13. Cook for more 1 minute as you keep stirring constantly.
14. Introduce the tomatoes.
15. Increase the heat to high, add the chickpeas.

16. Bring the mixture to a simmer, fluctuate the heat as required for 10 minutes.
17. Season to taste with additional salt or accordingly.
18. Serve over basmati rice and garnish with lemon wedges.
19. Enjoy.

Lemon green pasta with peas and ricotta

This lemon green pasta taste as delicious as its looks tempts your appetite. It is easier made with vegetables and herbs especially kale. Pasta and peas are all cooked in the same one pot.

Ingredients

- 1 large bunch of kale
- 2 large cloves garlic, smashed and peeled
- ¾ cup of coarsely grated Parmesan cheese
- ½ cup of ricotta cheese
- Zest and juice from 1 medium lemon
- ¼ teaspoon red pepper flakes
- Sea salt
- ¼ cup extra-virgin olive oil
- Freshly ground black pepper
- ½ pound of rigatoni or pappardelle
- 2 cups of fresh or frozen peas

Directions

1. Bring a large pot of salted water to boil.
2. As the water boils, prepare your kale by slicing, throw the rough bottom of the stems.
3. Slice the stems into pieces ¼-inch wide.
4. Place the stem pieces in a fine-mesh sieve.
5. When the water is ready, place the sieve in the water, resting the lip against the top of the pot.
6. Cook for 3 minutes, then remove the sieve and add all of the kale leaves to the pot.
7. Put the sieve back in the water on top of the leaves and cook for 5 minutes
8. Warm the olive oil in a small skillet over medium temperature.
9. Add the garlic, cook until the garlic begins to sizzle
10. Reduce the heat let simmer as you keep shimmying the pan and turning the garlic every constantly in 5 minutes.
11. After the garlic softens, remove the skillet from the heat and pour into a blender.
12. Add the cooked kale stems to the blender.
13. Add most of the zest from the lemon with 1 tablespoon of the juice.
14. Add ¼ teaspoon of salt, the red pepper flakes.
15. Blend until the mixture is completely smooth.
16. Taste and season accordingly. Set aside.

17. Cook the pasta as directed on the package. Make sure to keep of its boiling water as you drain out.
18. Return to the pot.
19. Pour in the green sauce, ¾ of the Parmesan and peas.
20. Add a small splash of the reserved cooking water stir to coat the pasta and bright green.
21. Divide into bowls.
22. Top each with a sprinkle of the remaining Parmesan, a few dollops of ricotta, and a sprinkle of lemon zest and red pepper flakes (optional).
23. Finish the bowls with a light drizzle of olive oil.
24. Serve and enjoy.

Best stuffed shells

Spinach and ricotta filling are stuffed in shells with the capacity of 8 servings, the recipe is quite delicious with cheesy saucy shells for dinner and lunch.

Ingredients

- 4 cloves garlic, peeled and cut into several segments
- Fresh basil for garnish
- ounces of grated part-skim mozzarella
- Freshly ground pepper
- 1 pound of fresh baby spinach
- ounces of ricotta cheese
- ounces of jumbo shells
- ½ teaspoon of red pepper flakes
- ¾ teaspoon of sea salt
- 1 tablespoon of extra virgin olive oil
- ¼ cup of chives or green onions
- 1 large egg
- ½ cup of grated Parmesan
- 3 cups of marinara sauce

Directions

1. Preheat your oven to 375°F with racks in the middle and upper third of the oven.

2. Bring a large stockpot of salted water to boil over high heat.

3. Add fresh greens to the boiling water, cook until wilted within 20 – 40 seconds.

4. Move the greens to the ice bath let cool.

5. Drain off the water in the greens keep aside for later

6. Bring the water in the pot back to a boil.

7. Gently add the pasta shells.

8. Cook until pliable in 10 minutes stir often.

9. Drain off the water, return the noodles to the pot.

10. Gently stir in the olive oil and keep aside.

11. Turn on your food processor and drop the garlic through the feeding tube.

12. When the garlic is chopped, stop the machine and scrape down the sides.

13. Add the greens to the bowl.

14. Process until the greens are chopped into small pieces.

15. Add the ricotta blended well.

16. Add half of the mozzarella, parmesan and chives, black pepper, red pepper flakes and salt, blend well.

17. Taste and season accordingly.

18. Add the eggs blended completely, also keep aside for later.

19. Spread 1 cup of the marinara sauce across the bottom.

20. Stuff each shell with a spoonful of the green mixture.

21. Place stuffed shells in the baker in rows.

22. Spoon the remaining marinara sauce over the tops of the shells.

23. Top with the remaining mozzarella.

24. Cover the baker with a foil let bake on the middle rack for 30 minute

25. Transfer the foil on the upper rack.

26. Bake for 5 – 10 minutes ensure the mozzarella is fully melted.

27. Garnish the shells with a grated parmesan and small fresh basil leaves.

28. Serve and enjoy.

Mango yogurt popsicles

This is per harps the most refreshing Mediterranean Sea diet healthiest mango drink with simple and easy to make ingredients. It is also perfect for the summer.

Ingredients

- 1 stick of unsalted butter
- 5 ounces of milk chocolate
- 1 cup of Greek yogurt
- 1 wedge lemon
- 1/4 cup of granulated sugar
- 2½ cups of frozen mango pieces, slightly thawed

Directions

1. Combine the yogurt together with lemon juice, sugar, and mango pieces in a food processor.
2. Process until smooth.
3. Pour the mixture in a popsicle mold with inserted sticks.
4. Place in the freezer overnight.
5. Remove the popsicles, allow then to heat to room temperature for a few minutes.

6.   Take out of the molds.

7.   Place a sheet of parchment paper in the freezer and place the popsicles onto it.

8.   Cut the chocolate into tiny pieces, place all of them a dish.

9.   Add diced butter and melt over a double boiler.

10. Pour this melted chocolate into mug that is preferably heat proof for dipping each popsicle.

11. As you take out, allow the excess chocolate to gently drip back.

12. Make sure to repeat this very step with all the reaming popsicles.

13. Place the ready ones back in the freezer.

14. Remove, let settle to a bit.

15. Serve and enjoy.

Banana bread

Banana is a fruit of the heart blessed with abundant fiber. Above and beyond, it is moist, soft and sweet. It is best with honey or butter depending on how you like it.

Ingredients

- A few drops of vanilla essence
- ½ cup of granulated sugar
- 1 large egg
- 1½ cup of all-purpose flour
- 1 teaspoon of baking soda
- 3 large ripe bananas
- ⅓ cup of unsalted butter
- 1 teaspoon of ground cinnamon

Directions

1. Begin by preparing the bananas, cut them into small pieces.
2. Put them in a medium sized dish, then mash them with a fork.
3. Add in large egg, beaten with a fork. Mix properly.
4. Add baking soda along with the melted butter, caster sugar, vanilla essence, flour. Make sure you mix well.

5. Pour the batter into a loaf tin lined with baking paper.

6. Place in a preheated oven and bake for 1 hour at 355°F.

7. Serve and enjoy.

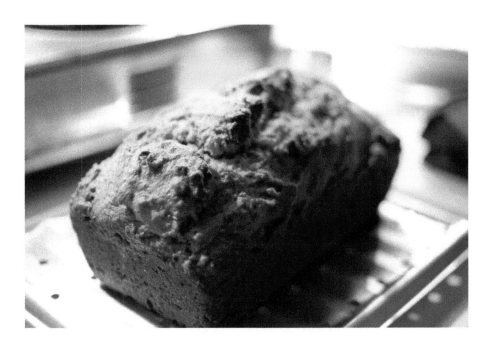

Chocolate Nutella mousse with strawberries

This is a desert with an exciting tasty and sweetness for any occasion. It is easy and quick to make in only 30 minutes, you will be exciting your taste buds with this Mediterranean Sea diet recipe.

Ingredients

- 2 tablespoons of lemon juice
- 2 cups of whipping cream
- 2 tablespoons of caster sugar
- 7 ounces of dark chocolate
- 2 cups of fresh strawberries
- 2 tablespoons of powdered sugar
- 5 tablespoons of Nutella

Directions

1. Start by cutting the chocolate into small pieces.
2. Over double boiler melt the chocolates with ½ cup of whipping cream. Allow it to cool.

3. As the chocolate melts, whip the cream together with the powdered sugar until soft peaks form.

4. Then, whisk Nutella with a few tablespoons of whipped cream in a large mixing dish.

5. Fold the whipped cream into the Nutella mixture.

6. It is time to stir in the cooled chocolate.

7. Divide the mousse into 5 glasses or more.

8. Place in the refrigerator for 60 minutes.

9. As the mousse refrigerates, prepare the strawberries by cleaning, and trimming any green parts.

10. Cut into small pieces.

11. Shift them into a bowl.

12. Add caster sugar and lemon juice.

13. Place in a refrigerator 30 minutes.

14. Remove and top each glass with strawberries and the juice if any.

15. Serve and enjoy.

No bake pineapple cake with Nutella

This incredible desert recipe only features 7 ingredients and gets ready in 20 minutes; a very short time, isn't it? This recipe can be made ahead of time with Nutella and pineapple pieces.

Ingredients

- 1 can of pineapple slices
- 1 ½ cup of sour cream
- 4 tablespoons of Nutella
- 2 tablespoons of powdered sugar
- ½ cup of Greek yogurt
- ½ cup of sour cream
- 3 tablespoons of powdered sugar
- 2 cups of graham crumbs, heaped
- ⅓ cup of unsalted butter

Directions

1. Mix melted butter together with the digestive biscuit crumbs. Endeavor to combine well.

2. Shift the entire mixture into cake tin, press down to make the crust.

3. Drain the pineapple slices of any excess unwanted water and pat them dry.

4. Cut 4 – 5 pineapple slices in halves.

5. Place them inside the cake pan with others (they should be separate; they should touch each other).

6. Any remaining pineapples should be cut into small pieces and spread them over the biscuit layer.

7. Whisk together powdered sugar with Nutella and the Sour cream to combined.

8. Spread this mixture over the pineapple slices.

9. Now, in another separate mixing dish, mix sour cream together with the powdered sugar, and Greek yogurt.

10. Spread over Nutella layer.

11. Cover this mixture with cling film.

12. Move it to the fridge, let refrigerate for at 14 hours.

13. You can beautify with pineapples if you like.

14. Serve and enjoy.

Strawberry marshmallow brownies

These Mediterranean Sea diet strawberry marshmallow brownies are chewy on the inside. They are delicious and can make a whole breakfast or as a desert.

Ingredients

- 4 Medium Eggs
- 7 ounces of Marshmallows
- 2 cups of Fresh Strawberries
- 7 ounces of Bittersweet
- 3/4 cup of Granulated Sugar
- 2 teaspoon of Baking Powder
- 11/4 cup of All-Purpose Flour
- 1½ stick of Unsalted Butter

Directions

1. Melt the chocolate with butter in a pot containing simmering water.
2. Allow it to cool when melted.

3.   Meanwhile, in a large bowl, whisk eggs, then add sugar. Continue to whisk until foamy.

4.   Adding in flour with the baking powder.

5.   Mix until smooth.

6.   Now, add melted chocolate mix to combined.

7.   Pour this mixture into a large baking pan that is well aligned with baking paper parchment.

8.   Then, bake for 10 minutes in a preheated oven at 360°F.

9.   Top with marshmallows together with the strawberries when the 10 minutes have run out.

10. Then move it back in the oven in the same pan.

11. Continue to bake another 10 minutes.

12. Serve and enjoy when ready.

Fried battered apple rings

This is a simple recipe to make in 5 minutes yet delicious and mouth-watering. Here, apple slices are simply dipped into batter, later deep fried and coated with some cinnamon sugar. It is a wonderful Mediterranean recipe to try at home.

Ingredients

- 11/4 cup of vegetable oil
- ½ cup of all-purpose flour
- 3 tablespoons of milk
- 1 teaspoon of ground cinnamon
- 1/4 cup of granulated sugar
- 1 teaspoon of rum
- 2 large apples
- 1 large egg
- 1 tablespoon of granulated sugar

Directions

1. Firstly, combine and mix flour together with the milk, rum, egg, sugar until smooth batter in a soup dish.
2. Clean and slice apples into thin slices with the core removed.

3.   Next, heat up oil in a frying pan until shimmering without smoke.

4.   Get every ring and dip in the batter and fry until all sides turn to golden brown.

5.   Fry all the 12 apple slices the same way in 5 minutes or so.

6.   Drain any excess oil with a kitchen towel.

7.   Coat in cinnamon sugar before they have cooled completely.

8.   Serve and enjoy.

Strawberry banana frozen yogurt

The Mediterranean Sea diet has invented many substitutions to consumption of unhealthy foods. This strawberry banana frozen yogurt is a perfect replacement for ice cream that has high sugar and calorie content.

Ingredients

- 2 tablespoon of honey
- 2 ripe bananas
- Frozen strawberries
- Greek yogurt

Directions

1. Firstly, place the strawberries to thaw a bit.
2. Then puree in a food processor.
3. Place in the peeled and sliced bananas to the mixture.
4. Add the yogurt to the mixture continue to process until smooth.
5. Taste and adjust accordingly.

6.   Transfer into a plastic container when tightly covered with a lid.
7.   Place in freezer and let freeze.
8.   Remove the container after 2 hours.
9.   Break the ice with a spoon.
10.   Serve and enjoy with your required consistency.

Mediterranean breakfast board

This particular Mediterranean diet is quite satisfying and wholesome. It features falafel, hummus, tabouli among others. Variety of vegetables are all blended in this recipe making it vegetarian.

Ingredients

- Fresh herbs for garnish
- 1 Baba Ganoush Recipe
- Feta cheese
- 1 Tabbouleh
- Marinated artichokes
- 1 to 2 tomatoes, sliced
- Pita Bread, sliced into quarters
- 1 Falafel Recipe
- 6 to 7 Radish, halved or sliced
- Assorted olives
- 1 Classic Hummus Recipe
- Extra virgin olive oil
- Grapes
- 1 English cucumber, sliced

Directions

1. Firstly, begin by making the falafel normally. Just make early enough.

2. Then make the hummus, baba ganoush normally. If possible, prepare all these components a head of time.

3. Next, slice the feta cheese.

4. Make tabbouleh normally. You can refrigerate if you made it couple of days earlier.

5. Place the hummus, baba ganoush, olive oil , tabbouleh in dishes.

6. Place the largest bowl in the center of a large wooden board as a focal point.

7. Arrange the remaining bowls on different parts of the board for easy movement as well as shape.

8. Any remaining ingredients should be obtained using the gap left between the bowls.

9. These ingredients are mainly vegetables and salads.

10. You can add grapes and garnish with fresh herbs.

11. Serve and enjoy.

Cinnamon walnut apple cake baked with olive oil

Ingredients

- 3 tablespoons of sesame seeds
- 1 cup of extra virgin olive oil
- 1 cup of brown sugar
- 2 ½ cups of wheat flour
- 2 teaspoons of baking powder
- 1 teaspoon of vanilla extract
- 4 apples, peeled, halved, cored, thinly sliced
- 4 eggs
- ½ cup of walnuts, chopped
- ½ cup of raisins
- 1 cup of milk
- 1 ½ teaspoons of ground cinnamon

Directions

1. Firstly, preheat your oven ready to 375°F.
2. Beat eggs and sugar with a hand mixer for 10 minutes.
3. Add olive oil continue to beat for 3 minutes.
4. Add milk together with baking powder, wheat flour, and vanilla.

5. Beat again for more 2 minutes.
6. Oil your cake pan then, add half the butter to your pan.
7. In a bowl, mix the apples together with brown sugar, raisins, walnuts, and cinnamon.
8. Pour the mixture on top of batter place in cake pan.
9. Add remaining batter to pan then sprinkle with sesame seeds.
10. Let bake for 45 – 50 minutes.
11. Serve (slice) and enjoy.

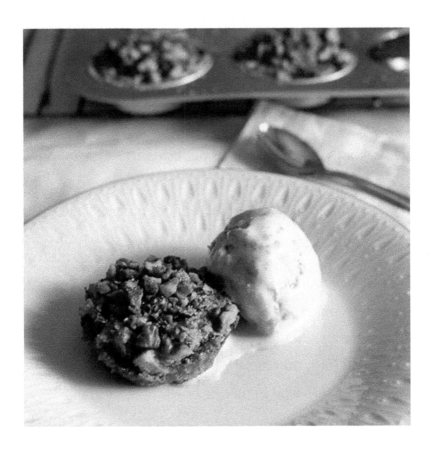

Anatolian flat bread with spinach and cheese

Ingredients

- 1 tablespoon of extra virgin olive oil
- 1 packet of instant dry yeast
- 3 tablespoons of extra virgin olive oil
- 1 lb. of all-purpose flour
- 1 cup of feta cheese
- 1 ½ cups of warm water
- 1 cup of baby spinach
- 1 onion, finely chopped
- 2 tablespoons of plain yogurt
- Pinch of salt
- 1 teaspoon of Turkish red pepper flakes

Directions

1. Start by combining cup of warm water, yeast, and a pinch of salt in a small sized mixing bowl, stir to dissolve completely.
2. Let rest for 5 minutes for bubbles to form on surface.
3. Transfer into a large mixing bowl.

4. Create a well in the middle for pouring in the yeast, yoghurt, olive oil, water salt mixture, and the balance of the warm water.

5. Immediately make a dough with your hand. Knead to form a soft dough.

6. Divide into 5 pieces, roll into balls.

7. Place the balls on a surface floured.

8. Cover with damp cloth let rest for 1 hour.

9. Chop the washed spinach leaves.

10. Knead the onions together with the spinach, olive oil, and red pepper flakes briefly.

11. Stir in the feta cheese and combine well.

12. Roll out the balls of the dough into thin, flat rounds.

13. Then, sprinkle a little flour as you roll the dough for all the balls.

14. Fold the top and bottom sides of the dough a way for the edges to meet in the middle.

15. Spread filling into the middle part of this flat sheet.

16. Then fold the right and left edges over the filling.

17. Press the edges together to seal. Do this for all the doughs.

18. Next, heat a pan and brush with some olive oil.

19. Cook for 2 – 3 minutes.

20. Brush the uncooked side with olive oil and flip over.

21. Let cook for 2 – 3 minutes

22. Cook the rest the same way.

Apple and carrot superhero muffins

The apple and carrot superhero muffins is a perfect Mediterranean Sea diet for breakfast. It is naturally a sweet and gluten free recipe with a heart apple and carrots.

Ingredients

- 6 tablespoons of unsalted butter, melted
- 1 ½ cups of old-fashioned oats
- 1 teaspoon of baking soda
- ½ teaspoon of fine sea salt
- ½ cup of chopped walnuts
- ½ cup of honey or maple syrup
- 2 cups of packed almond meal or almond flour
- 2 teaspoons of ground cinnamon
- 3 eggs
- 1 cup of grated Granny Smith apple
- 1 cup of peeled and grated carrots

Directions

1. Preheating your oven to 350°F ready is a perfect start.

2. Align a standard muffin tin with paper muffin cup in the oven.

3. In a large mixing bowl, combine almond meal together with the oats, baking soda, cinnamon, and salt

4. In another separate mixing bowl, whisk honey together with the eggs and butter.

5. Next, whisk grated apple and carrots place in.

6. Pour the mixture into the dry ingredients make sure they combine well.

7. Spoon the batter into the muffin cups, filling each to the brim.

8. Place in the oven and bake until the muffins turn to brown on top in 25 – 30 minutes.

9. Let cool totally.

10. Serve and enjoy.

Simple breakfast tostadas

In a total preparation and cook time of 40 minutes, you would have completed making your breakfast tostadas. This is typically a vegetarian breakfast recipe fit for a Mediterranean vegan.

Ingredients

- Avocado
- 1 tablespoon of extra-virgin olive oil
- 2 cups of refried beans , warmed
- ½ cup of grated sharp cheddar cheese
- 8 corn tortillas
- Salsa
- 2 cups of Pico de Gallo
- 8 eggs, fried or scrambled

Directions

1. Preheat your oven to 400°F.
2. Align your baking oven with 2 large baking sheets with parchment paper.
3. Brush both sides of the tortilla with oil.
4. Organize 4 tortillas in a single layer across every baking pan.

5. Then, bake while turning half way for 10 – 12 minutes till golden.

6. Prepare the remaining components especially the Pico de Gallo, eggs, and beans accordingly.

7. Spread the tostada with warm refried beans.

8. Use the cheese for topping along with egg. Except top the eggs with Pico de Gallo.

9. Serve and enjoy.

Avocado toast

Avocados are known to be a healthy remedy for nourishing the skin. As a result, make this Mediterranean Sea diet the number one on your diet to witness some glittering skin on your body. It is a satisfying crisp cream. It is largely a snack.

Ingredients

- ½ ripe avocado
- Pinch of salt
- 1 slice of bread

Directions

1. Begin by toasting the slice of bread to your liking.
2. Cut and remove pit from the avocado.
3. Scoop all the flesh in a bowl and easily smash with the back of your spoon till very smooth
4. Mix in a pinch of salt.
5. Spread avocado on top of your toast.
6. Enjoy.

Creamiest scrambled eggs with goat cheese

Ingredients

- 3 cups of baby spinach, roughly chopped
- ⅓ cup of whole milk or milk of choice
- ⅓ cup of oil-packed sun-dried tomatoes, rinsed, chopped
- Freshly ground black pepper
- 4 ounces of goat cheese, crumbled
- Pinch of fine sea salt
- 1 tablespoon of unsalted butter
- 8 large eggs
- ½ cup of chopped green onion, mostly green parts

Directions

1. Begin by crack your eggs into a large bowl.
2. Add milk, salt, and black pepper.
3. Then, whisk to combined the mixture. It should be a pure yellow.
4. Warm a medium skillet over medium heat.
5. Melt in some bit of butter.

6. Then proceed to add spinach let cook for 2 minutes as you stir till the spinach is wilted.

7. Pour the eggs into the skillet immediately lower the heat.

8. Stir the eggs gently with a spatula until clumpy in 4 – 5 minutes.

9. Take off heat source.

10. Add the goat cheese together with the green onion and sun-dried tomatoes, stir to combine.

11. Divide into bowls.

12. Sprinkle with topping of your choice.

13. Serve and enjoy.

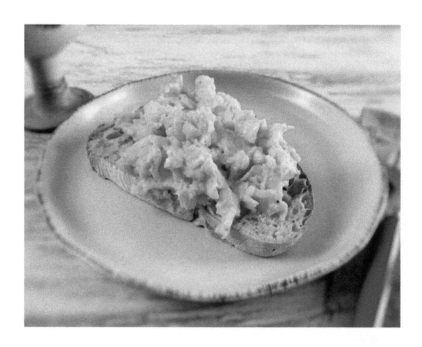

Strawberry oat muffins

These fruity strawberry muffins originate from the idea of Mediterranean Sea diet of consuming only vegetables, fruits and any other natural foods. The strawberry is made with whole grains rich in carbohydrates for breakfast.

Ingredients

- 1 teaspoon of turbinado sugar
- 2 cups of hulled and diced ripe strawberries
- ⅓ cup of old-fashioned oats
- 2 teaspoons of vanilla extract
- ½ teaspoon of fine sea salt
- ⅓ cup of extra-virgin olive oil
- ⅓ cup of maple syrup
- 2 eggs at room temperature
- ½ teaspoon of baking soda
- 1 cup of plain Greek yogurt
- 1 3/4 cups of white whole wheat flour
- 1 teaspoon of baking powder

Directions

1. Preheat the oven to 400° F.

2. Combine flour together with the oats, baking soda, baking powder, and salt in a large mixing bowl. Whisk to blend.

3. In a separate medium mixing dish, combine oil with maple syrup and eggs. Beat thoroughly together and whisk.

4. Add yogurt with vanilla to the mixture and blend further.

5. Mix the wet ingredients with the dry ones, blend well to combine.

6. Next is to carefully fold the strawberries into the batter.

7. Distribute the batter equally in all the 12 muffin cups.

8. Sprinkle the tops with oats and turbinado sugar.

9. Place in the oven let bake for 19 – 22 minutes.

10. Let the muffins cool on a rack.

11. Enjoy your deliciously healthy breakfast.

2   821. Breakfast quesadillas

3   The actual cook time for this flavorful delicious quesadilla is just 10 minutes. It features scrambled eggs, herbs, beans for a healthy breakfast. It is protein rich; therefore, your protein needs are sorted.

4   Ingredients

1. In a bowl, whisk eggs with the hot sauce and salt until blended.

2. Introduce the beans to the mixture and keep for later.

3. In a medium-sized skillet melt the butter over medium heat until bubbling.

4. Pour in the egg mixture and cook for 3 minutes max as you stir.

5. Shift the whole mixture to a bowl.

6. Stir in the green onion together with the cilantro and jalapeño.

7. In another separate large skillet, warm the tortilla over medium temperature, keep flipping infrequently.

8. After they have warmed, sprinkle one-half of the cheese over one-half of the tortilla.

9. Top scrambled eggs on the cheese. Then with the balance of the cheese.

10. Evenly press the empty tortilla halve over the toppings.

11. Place on heat, let cook until golden in 2 minutes. Repeat this step for both sides of the tortilla.

12. Transfer the quesadilla to a chopping board, allow it to cool.

13. Slice and enjoy for breakfast.

Mediterranean breakfast strata

Ingredients

- Kosher salt
- 2 shallots minced
- 4 ounces of Ciliegine Fresh Mozzarella cheese balls halved
- 1 cup of button mushrooms sliced
- 1 teaspoon of dried marjoram leaves
- 1/4 cup of shredded Parmesan cheese plus additional for topping
- 6 cups of white bread cut into ½ inch chunks
- 1/4 cup of basil leaves slivered
- ½ cup of artichoke hearts cut into 1/8ths
- 3 tablespoons of butter
- 1/4 cup of Kalamata olives quartered
- 1 ½ cups of half and half
- 1/4 cup of marinated sun dried tomatoes slivered
- 2 cloves garlic minced
- 6 eggs

Directions

1. Begin by melting 1 tablespoon of butter.

2. Then, preheat your oven to 325°F.

3. In large skillet over medium heat, melt remaining 2 tablespoons of butter.

4. Add garlic and shallot let sauté for 2 minutes.

5. Add mushrooms and marjoram let cook for more 4 minutes.

6. Remove from heat source and place mushroom mixture in large bowl with bread chunks, Kalamata olives, sun dried tomatoes, Parmesan artichoke hearts, and Fresh Mozzarella and stir to mix.

7. Season lightly with kosher salt.

8. Fill baking dishes evenly with the bread mixture.

9. In 4-cup liquid measuring cup, mix eggs with half and half and pour 1 cup of egg mixture evenly over bread in each dish.

10. Garnish with basil and Parmesan.

11. Place baking dishes on a baking sheet.

12. Let bake for 50 minutes until eggs have set.

13. Remove from oven and let settle for 5 minutes.

14. Serve and enjoy.

Gluten-free pumpkin oat pancakes

In an equivalent of 25 minutes you can have your nutritious and healthy pumpkin oat pancakes ready for your bite. As long as the pumpkins cook over low heat and slow, you will have a tasty delicious meal very fluffy and easy to bite.

Ingredients

- ½ teaspoon of ground ginger
- 1 cup of oat flour
- 1 cup of pumpkin puree
- 1/4 teaspoon of ground nutmeg
- 1/4 cup of milk of choice
- ½ teaspoon of baking soda
- 2 tablespoons of coconut oil melted
- 1 tablespoon of lemon juice
- ½ teaspoon of salt
- 1 teaspoon of maple syrup
- 1/4 teaspoon of ground cloves or allspice
- ½ teaspoon of ground cinnamon
- 1 teaspoon of vanilla extract
- 2 eggs

Directions

1. In a small mixing bowl, stir together the pumpkin puree with lemon juice, coconut oil, milk, maple syrup, and vanilla.
2. Beat in the eggs.
3. In a medium sized bowl, whisk the oat flour together with baking soda, salt and spices.
4. Form a well in the center of the dry ingredients.
5. In the well, pour in the wet ingredients.
6. With a big spoon, stir the dry ingredients are thoroughly until moistened.
7. Let the batter to settle for 10 minutes.
8. Heat a heavy cast iron skillet over medium-low temperature.
9. Lightly oil the surface of your pan with coconut oil.
10. Pour 1/4 cup of batter onto the pan.
11. Place the pancake let cook for 3 minutes, until bubbles begin to form around the edges.
12. Flip it with a spatula when it turns golden continue to cook for more 1 minute and 30 seconds until golden brown on every sides.
13. Serve the pancakes immediately
14. And enjoy.

Gingerbread granola

Ginger is famous for a vibrantly delicious taste and aroma in whatever dish it features in. As such, the granola is irresistibly spiced with ginger and cinnamon to tease your taste buds and keep you hooked to eating more and more. Maple dry syrup is ultimately used to sweeten it up.

Ingredients

- 1 teaspoon of vanilla extract
- 1 ½ cups of raw pecans and/or walnuts
- 1 teaspoon of ground ginger
- ⅓ cup of real maple syrup
- 1 teaspoon of fine-grain sea salt
- ⅓ cup of chopped candied ginger
- 1 teaspoon of ground cinnamon
- ⅓ cup of chopped dried cranberries
- 1/4 cup of molasses
- ½ cup of melted coconut oil
- ½ cup of large, unsweetened coconut flakes
- 4 cups of old-fashioned rolled oats

Directions

1. Begin by preheating your oven to 350°F.

2. Align a half-sheet pan with parchment paper in the oven.

3. In a large sized mixing bowl, combine nuts, the oats, cinnamon, salt, and ground ginger stir well to allow it to combine.

4. Stir in the oil, molasses, maple syrup, and vanilla.

5. Move the granola out onto the prepared pan and.

6. With a big spoon, spread it evenly to form a layer.

7. Bake for 10 minutes in the preheated oven.

8. Remove from the oven to top with coconut flakes.

9. Stir up the mixture to ensure balanced cooked granola.

10. Return the pan to the oven for 10 or more minutes accordingly.

11. Top the granola with the chopped cranberries and candied ginger.

12. Allow it to cool off.

13. Break them into pieces. Enjoy.

14. Store the granola in an airtight container.

15. It can stay fresh for 1 or 2 weeks if properly refrigerated.

Broiled grapefruit with honey yogurt and granola

In 20 minutes, this recipe will be ready to kill your hunger and satisfy your taste buds. Served with yogurt and granola substance, this recipe uses grapefruits sprinkled with sugar.

Ingredients

- Granola
- Greek yogurt or thick goat's yogurt
- 6 tablespoons of raw sugar or brown sugar
- Sprinkle ground ginger
- Dash sea salt
- Sprinkle ground cinnamon
- 3 grapefruits
- Honey

Directions

1. Firstly, preheat broiler.
2. Make the bases of your grapefruit halves flat.
3. Slice off 1/4-inch of the peel on the base end and the stem end of each grapefruit.

4. Slice each grapefruit in half but parallel to the initial cuts.

5. Place the halved grapefruits face-down on paper towels for 5 minutes in order to absorb excess moisture form the grapefruit.

6. In a small sized bowl, mix the raw or brown sugar together with a sprinkle of ginger and cinnamon do not forget to add a dash of salt.

7. Get a rimmed baking sheet then place the grapefruit halves face up.

8. Using 1 tablespoon per half, sprinkle each halve with the sugar mixture.

9. Proceed to broil for 7 – 10 minutes or till the sugar has melted

10. Allow the grapefruits to cool for 3 or so minutes.

11. Serve warm with a big dollop of yogurt and with the handful of granola.

2 Enjoy.

Vegetarian fresh spring rolls with peanut sauce

Using peanut butter as a dipping option for the vegetable spring rolls makes this recipe quite unique. The raw veggies are boosted by the salty feta cheese with its great aromatic refreshing healthy flavor.

Ingredients

- Feta cheese
- 2 medium carrots
- 1 teaspoon of soy sauce
- 1 large yellow/red bell pepper
- 2 cups of baby kale leaves
- ¼ head of purple cabbage
- 2 tablespoons of water
- 2 medium avocados
- 4 tablespoons of peanut butter
- 1 small lemon
- 2 tablespoons of honey
- 6 rice paper sheets

Directions

1. Prepare the veggies by cutting the pepper and carrots into matchsticks.
2. Slice avocados and cabbage as thinly.
3. Remove any hard stems from baby kale leaves.
4. In a large frying pan, place warm water in to soak the rice paper until soft in about 20 seconds or more.
5. Remove when the rice paper has completely softened when felt.
6. Place the soften paper onto a clean work top and add the fillings beginning at the bottom ⅓ of the paper.
7. Crumble some Feta cheese over it, add some carrots, peppers, and cabbage.
8. Roll the fillings in the paper as if you are wrapping. Nevertheless, only roll to close the first batch.
9. Add more fillings mainly the avocado and the kale, once you have finished rolling.
10. Hold the fillings with your hands as you roll the roll away while tucking the fillings in.
11. Close both edges by folding the rice paper in and complete the rolling.
12. Keep pressing the roll to ensure the fillings are not loose.
13. Combine all the ingredients until smooth, for the peanut butter after softening in a microwave.
14. Serve immediately and enjoy.

Cheese tortellini pasta with broccoli and bacon

Just reserve 20 minutes to complete making this cheese tortellini pasta with broccoli and bacon using only 5 ingredients.

Ingredients

- 16 ounces of fresh cheese tortellini
- 1 cup of single cream
- 2 cups of bacon slices (200 grams)
- 2 cups of cheddar cheese or similar, grated
- 2 cups of broccoli florets

Directions

1. Boil a large pot of water.
2. Throw in tortellini and broccoli.
3. Cook until ready in 5 minutes or according to the package instruction of the tortellini.
4. Fry the bacon.
5. Pour in cream as you stir.
6. Reduce the heat as the sauce thickens, stir in grated cheese.

7. Turn off the source of heat.

8. Drain excess water in the tortellini and broccoli.

9. Pour the cheesy bacon sauce over and mix

10. Serve warm and enjoy with cheese though optional.

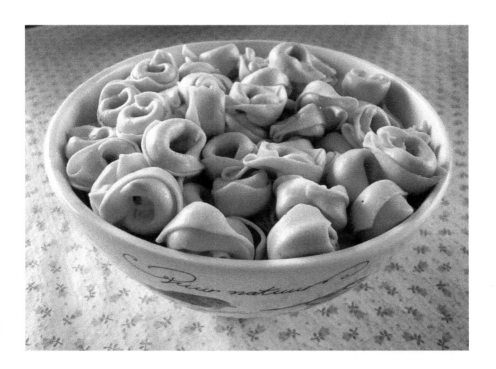

Simple campfire stew

If you have a crowd to feed do not look further. Here is the right recipe to handle a crowd.

Ingredients

- 3 tablespoon of Salt
    - lb. of Boston Butt or Pork Shoulder
- lb. of Potatoes
- 4.5 lb. of Beef Round Steak
- tablespoon of Dried Marjoram
- 11 cups of Water
- Dried of Fresh Chili Pepper, optional
- Garlic Cloves
- 1 can of Beer
- ½ cup of Lard
- tablespoon of Caraway Seeds
- 1½ lb. of Onion
- 2½ tablespoon of Sweet Paprika
- 1 tablespoon of Tomato Paste

Directions

1. In large pot, melt the lard.
2. Add diced onion and sauté for 5 minutes.
3. Add the meats diced into small pieces.
4. Let them brown as you stir occasionally.
5. Add sweet paprika, toss to mix well, let cook for 1 minute.
6. Add 4 cups water, caraway seeds, salt, ½ of diced potatoes, and 1 can of beer.
7. Cover with lid tightly let cook as you keep checking once in a time.
8. Keep checking the amount of water, add accordingly, continue to simmer for 1 hour and 30 minutes then add the rest of the potatoes, add water accordingly.
9. Cook until the meat is ready.
10. Add the tomato paste, marjoram, minced garlic, and dried whole chili, when the meat is about to get ready to flavor it.
11. Taste and season accordingly.
12. Serve when warm with slices of bread.
13. Enjoy.

Spicy spaghetti aglio olio and pepperoncino

Ingredients

- Chili
- 1 cup of parmesan cheese, grated
- 5 - 6 tablespoon of extra virgin olive oil
- 1 pounds Spaghetti
- 2 cups of fresh flat leaf parsley, chopped
- 10 - 12 cloves Garlic
- Salt

Directions

1. Start off with boiling water for spaghetti.
2. When the water is boiling, add salt and spaghetti cook as instructed on the package by the manufacturer
3. As the spaghetti is boiling, rinse parsley and chili.
4. Chop all of them finely.
5. Peel and thinly chop garlic.
6. Grate Parmesan.
7. When the spaghetti is about to get ready, heat oil in a frying pan.

8. Add garlic, sauté for 2 minutes on low temperature while stirring infrequently.
9. place in the parsley together with the chili and some tablespoons of pasta water allow it cook for 2 minutes.
10. Drain spaghetti of excess water and pour the sauce over it.
11. Sprinkle with Parmesan
12. Serve and enjoy.

Cauliflower bake with blue cheese and prosciutto

This recipe turns the ordinary veggie to something remarkably delicious using as an appetizer with blue cheese.

Ingredients

- 3 carrots
- 1 egg
- 4 tablespoon of olive oil
- 1 small onion, diced
- 4 prosciutto
- 1 pounds of cauliflower
- 2 tablespoons of bread crumbs
- ¼ cup of fresh flat leaf parsley, finely chopped
- Salt and pepper
- ¼ cup of blue cheese

Instruction

1. Wash the carrots well, peel and grate.
2. Secondly, wash the cauliflower, remove any green parts.
3. Chop into smaller pieces

4. Place in food processor, process until crumb like texture forms.
5. In a large bowl, blend processed cauliflower, carrots, diced onion, seasoning, breadcrumbs and the egg.
6. In a frying pan, heat the oil and sauté the cauliflower mixture for 5 minutes, keep stirring occasionally.
7. Stir in the fresh parsley.
8. Line a square sandwich pan with baking parchment paper.
9. Fill the bottom with half of the cauliflower mixture.
10. Push it down with the back of a spoon.
11. Add prosciutto torn into smaller pieces together with the crumbled cheese.
12. Cover tightly with the rest of the cauliflower mixture, again push it down to the bottom.
13. Now bake in already heated oven for 15 minutes.
14. Serve and enjoy as an appetizer or side dish.

Spinach crepes with pan-roasted vegetables

Ginger with its strong aromatic flavor is used for topping in this recipe with mushrooms, pepper, tomatoes and onions in 30 minutes of total preparation time. It is perfect for diner, lunch and even breakfast.

Ingredients

- 1 cup of milk
- 1 cup of plain flour
- 1 teaspoon pink Himalayan salt
- ½ teaspoon of pink Himalayan salt
- 1 thumb-size piece of fresh ginger, grated
- 1 cup of grated cheese of your choice
- 3 tablespoons of butter
- 2 cups of chopped mushrooms
- 1 yellow bell pepper
- 4 cups of fresh spinach
- 1 medium onion
- 2 cups of cherry tomatoes
- 2 cups of chopped flat leaf parsley
- 1 cup of grated cheese of your choice

- 1 tablespoon dried oregano
- 1 large egg
- 3 garlic cloves
- Sunflower oil for frying

Directions

1. In a food processor, blend the spinach together with the milk until smooth.
2. Pour the mixture in a bowl.
3. Add flour, egg, salt, and grated ginger, then whisk till well combined.
4. Heat up the frying pan.
5. Add a little oil and place in the batter.
6. Spread around evenly
7. Once set, turn it over and cook for 1 minute.
8. Melt the butter in a frying pan.
9. Add sliced mushrooms, onion, and pepper.
10. Roast for 10 minutes then add the cherry tomatoes together with garlic.
11. Continue to roast for more 2 – 3 minutes.
12. Switch off the heat.
13. Stir in the parsley.
14. Fill pancakes with vegetable mixture.
15. Sprinkle with grated cheese.
16. Serve when warm and enjoy.

Baked curry chicken wings with mango chutney

The mango chutney is used to perfectly marinate the chicken wings when are have become very tender and then baked for diner, lunch or breakfast

Ingredients

- ⅔ cup of mango chutney
- 2.5 pounds of chicken wings
- 4 tablespoons of curry powder
- 2 tablespoon of oyster sauce
- 2 2 tablespoon of Worcestershire sauce
- Teaspoons of pink Himalayan salt

Instruction

1. Place chicken wings in a bowl.
2. Season with salt and curry powder.
3. Mix well to ensure even coating.
4. In a separate bowl combine the Worcestershire sauce, mango chutney, and oyster sauce.

5. Pour gently over wings, mix until each piece is well coated in the sauce.
6. Cover the bowl with a close zip-lock bag and refrigerate for not less than 30 minutes.
7. After it is marinated, put the wings onto a baking tray lined with baking paperwith enough space between them.
8. Spoon the marinade over the wings.
9. Bake in a preheated oven at 200° for 25 minutes.
10. Serve and enjoy with a dip of your liking.

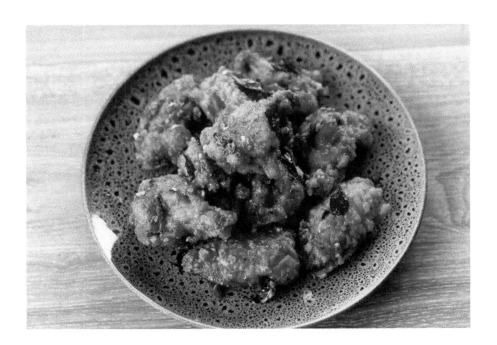

10-minute bake bean pasta sauce

Ingredients

- A handful of fresh flat leaf parsley
- 1 can of tomato pasta
- 1 can of baked beans in tomato sauce
- 3.5 oz. of cheddar cheese
- 3 garlic cloves
- 4.5 oz. of chorizo

Instruction

1. Begin by chop chorizo into smaller pieces.
2. Place in a frying pan do not add all oil because it has its own fat that will melt.
3. Peel and slice garlic cloves put to the chorizo.
4. Cook for 5 minutes as you stir occasionally.
5. Add the tomato pasta together with the baked beans.
6. Lower the heat let simmer for 5 minutes.
7. Put in the finely chopped parsley when it is about to get ready.
8. Turn off the heat and stir in cheese
9. Serve immediately with pasta.
10. Enjoy.

Sweet chili pesto burger sliders

This recipe combines sweet chili sauce, pesto, tomatoes, salad leaves and pesto burgers among other ingredients for a tasty breakfast to boost your healthy in 30 minutes' periods.

Ingredients

- Mixed salad leaves or lamb lettuce
- ¼ teaspoon of pink Himalayan salt
- 1 lb. of minced beef (440g)
- ¼ teaspoon of black pepper
- 9 mini burger buns
- 2 tomatoes
- 3 tablespoons of green pesto
- 2 tablespoons of pesto
- Sweet chili sauce to your taste
- 1 egg

Directions

1. In a bowl, mix pepper, salt, pesto, minced beef, and eggs.
2. Form into patties by rolling the mixture into a bowl, after which you flatten them, make less than 11 patties.

3. Place each patty on a baking tray lined with baking paper.
4. Move them to the oven heated to 190° and bake for 20 minutes.
5. Cut each bun in half.
6. Spread over with sweet chili sauce.
7. Add lamb lettuce together with tomato slice and a teaspoon of pesto.
8. Followed by burger patty and more lettuce.
9. Cover with bun.
10. Pierce with burger skewer.
11. Serve and enjoy.

Whole wheat crispy popcorn chicken wrap

Whole wheat as a food is a healthy and nutritious with high fiber and carbohydrate content to boost a person's energy. In this recipe, it is used to coat the chicken wrapped with veggies.

Ingredients

- ¼ cabbage
- 1 tomato
- 1 green bell pepper
- 1 romaine lettuce
- 6 whole wheat tortillas
- 7 ounces of popcorn chicken

Directions

1. Begin by rinsing the veggies under running water.
2. Thinly slice cabbage and so the romaine lettuce.
3. Dice tomatoes and peppers.
4. Place everything in a mixing bowl mix to combine.
5. Next, deep-fry the homemade popcorn chicken as per the manufacturer Directions.

6. Place tortilla onto a plate and spread the salad across the middle.
7. Add popcorn chicken and roll the tortilla over the filling to coat.
8. Cut in half and wrap in a piece of baking parchment.
9. Serve immediately and enjoy.

Nourishing Buddha bowl

Nourishing as the name suggests, this recipe is rich in nutrient though light meal. It only takes 25 minutes to get ready making it a quick meal which can also be prepared ahead.

Ingredients

- 1 baby romaine lettuce
- 6 tablespoons of natural yogurt or sour cream
- 1.7 ounces of buckwheat
- 2 tablespoons of unsalted butter
- 2 tablespoons of ketchup
- 2 avocados (medium)
- 2 spring onions (scallions)
- 2 carrots
- Drizzle of lemon juice
- 1 teaspoon of sweet paprika
- 3 ounces of chickpea cooked
- Drizzle of extra virgin olive oil
- ½-1 teaspoon of Himalayan salt to taste

Directions

1. Start by cooking the buckwheat as instructed by the manufacturer.
2. When ready, Season the water with ½ teaspoon salt.
3. As it cooks, rinse all the vegetables.
4. Peel and slice carrots.
5. Cut the spring onions and lettuce.
6. Cut avocado in half, remove the seed then scoop out using a spoon.
7. Cut it into strips
8. Melt the butter in a pan.
9. Add in drained chickpea let roast for 3 minutes.
10. Add sweet paprika toss around until all the chickpeas are coated evenly.
11. Continue to roast for more 2 minutes.
12. Turn off the heat.
13. Taste and season accordingly.
14. Arrange all the ingredients in a bowl, serve warm with a lemon wedge and extra virgin olive oil.
15. Enjoy.

Mini vegetarian puff pastry pizzas

The mini vegetarian puff pastry pizza will be ready in not more than 10 minutes topped with fresh vegetables and arugula as well as cheese.

Ingredients

- A handful of fresh arugula
- 1 batch homemade pizza sauce
- 6 cherry tomatoes, thinly sliced
- ½ small onion, thinly sliced
- 1 chili pepper, thinly sliced
- 6 olives, thinly sliced
- 1 puff pastry sheet
- 6 goat cheese, thin slices (optional)
- 1 small zucchini, sliced
- 1 ounce blue cheese

Directions

1. Preheat your oven to 200°.
2. As the oven heats, roll out the puff pastry sheet so thin.

3. Using a 4-inch round cookie cutter, cut out many circles.
4. Place them onto a baking tray lined with baking parchment.
5. Use an inch smaller cutter to make smaller circles inside the pastry, make sure not to cut through.
6. Top the pastry circles with a teaspoon of pizza sauce each piece, cherry tomatoes, some slices of zucchini, olives, little onion, and goat cheese and or blue cheese.
7. Sprinkle with chili pepper
8. Repeat this process and then bake at 200° for 10 – 15 minutes.
9. Top with arugula though optional but it is good.
10. Serve and enjoy.

Savory crepes with chia seeds and garlic

Savory crepes can be made nicely with minced meat with some canned tomatoes and variety of vegetables. Milk, rye and garlic with chia seeds elevate this recipe to the next level.

Ingredients

- ¼ tsp salt
- ½ cup rye flour
- 2 cups milk
- 1 tablespoon of dried oregano
- 1 tablespoon of chia seeds
- 3 cloves garlic
- ½ cup plain flour
- 1 medium egg

Directions

1. In a bowl, combine all the ingredients mix until you get a smooth batter
2. Heat a frying pan over a moderate temperature.
3. Add some oil in the pan.

4. Pour in the batter, then spread evenly by tilting the pan to all directions

5. Place in the pancakes until a visible golden brown color underneath.

6. Cook for more 1 – 2 minutes.

7. Move all to a plate when ready.

8. Serve and enjoy.

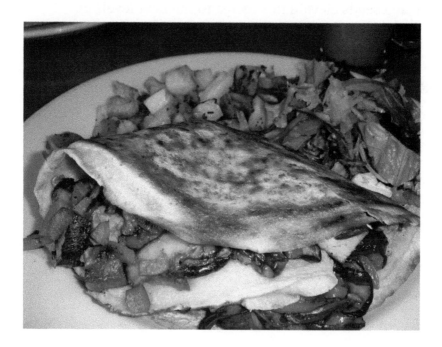

Panko salmon with snap peas

Prepared with Dijon mustard, this simple fresh tarragon kicks in with a sweet anise-y flavor. The salmon seared crusted side down is much easier to flip when golden and crispy. Snap peas are sweeter when crisp tender as this recipe just makes it.

Ingredients

- ½ tablespoon of Dijon mustard
- ½ teaspoon of canola mayonnaise
- ½ teaspoon of black pepper divided
- ¾ teaspoon of kosher salt
- 4 skinless of salmon fillets
- 1 tablespoon of chopped fresh tarragon
- ½ cup of whole wheat panko
- 2 teaspoons of grated lemon rind
- 2 tablespoon of olive oil
- 1/3 cup of thinly sliced shallots
- 2 teaspoon of fresh lemon juice
- 2 cups of sugar snap peas, trimmed

Directions

1 Start by combining mayonnaise, ½ teaspoon of salt, mustard, and ¼ teaspoon of pepper in a shallow bowl.

2 Spoon mustard mixture evenly over fillets.

3 Combine panko with 1 teaspoon of tarragon, and 1 teaspoon of the lemon rind in a bowl.

4 Sprinkle panko mixture over fillets ensure to press down to combine.

5 Heat 1 tablespoon of oil in a large skillet over medium temperature.

6 Add panko side down, fillets, to the heated pan let cook for 3 – 4 minutes

7 Turnover, continue to cook for more 3 – 4 minutes.

8 Remove from heat source and keep warm

9 Increase heat to high.

10 Add remaining 1 tablespoon of oil to pan.

11 Add snap peas and shallots let cook for 3 minutes as you keep stirring occasionally.

12 Add remaining ¼ teaspoon of salt, 1 teaspoon of lemon rind, ¼ teaspoon of pepper, ½ teaspoons of tarragon, and juice to pan

13 Let cook for 2 minutes until crisp-tender.

14 Serve with fillets.

15 Enjoy.

Arugula and cremini quiche with gluten-free almond meal crust

This is a gourmet simple recipe for any meal whether lunch, dinner or breakfast. It combines gluten-free thyme, almond meal crust, arugula and cremini mushrooms along with goat cheese to give a tasty feel in the taste buds.

Ingredients

- 5 ounces of goat cheese, crumbled
- 3 garlic cloves, pressed or minced
- 3 cups of baby arugula, roughly chopped
- 2 cups of packed almond meal or almond flour
- ⅓ cup of milk
- ¼ teaspoon of red pepper flakes
- ¼ teaspoon of freshly ground pepper
- 1 tablespoon of and 1 teaspoon water
- 1 ½ cups of cleaned and sliced Cremini mushrooms
- ⅓ cup of olive oil
- 1 teaspoon of salt
- Drizzle olive oil
- 6 large eggs
- 1 tablespoon of minced fresh thyme or 1 teaspoon dried thyme

Directions

1. Preheat oven to 400°F.
2. Oil a cast iron skillet with olive oil.

3. In a mixing bowl, stir together the garlic, thyme, almond meal, salt and pepper.
4. Pour in the olive oil and water, stir to combine them mixture.
5. Press the dough into your prepared skillet evenly across the bottom at least 1 ¼ inch up the sides.
6. Bake until the crust is lightly golden and firm to the touch in 15 – 20 minutes.
7. In a large oven at high temperature, warm enough olive oil to lightly coat the pan.
8. Cook the mushrooms with a dash of salt, stir often till it becomes tender.
9. Toss in the arugula and let it wilt, keep stirring for 30 seconds.
10. Move the mixture to a plate, let cool.
11. In another mixing bowl, whisk together the milk, eggs, salt and red pepper.
12. Gently stir in the goat cheese together with the slightly cooled mushroom and arugula mixture.
13. After baking the crust, pour in the egg mixture, let bake for 30 minutes.
14. Allow the quiche to cool for 5 or 10 minutes
15. Slice with a sharp knife.
16. Serve immediately and enjoy.

Huevos rancheros with avocado salsa Verde

Black beans together with fresh creamy avocado make this delicious rancheros recipe. It is healthy and tasty for a great dinner. Meatless but packed with veggies, this makes a great Mediterranean Sea diet.

Ingredients

- ½ lime, halved
- 1 tablespoon of olive oil
- ½ teaspoon of chili powder
- ¼ teaspoon of cayenne pepper
- 1 lime, halved
- ½ cup of feta, crumbled
- ½ jalapeño, seeds, membranes removed, finely chopped
- Salt and pepper
- 2 cans pf black black beans, rinsed and drained
- 1 cup of mild salsa Verde
- 4 or more eggs
- 1 ripe avocado, pitted and sliced
- ½ medium red onion, chopped
- 1 medium jalapeño, deseeded and roughly chopped

- 4 radishes, sliced into thin pieces
- Hot sauce
- 1 garlic clove, chopped
- 4 or more corn tortillas
- Big handful of cilantro
- Small handful cilantro, chopped
- ½ teaspoon of cumin powder

Directions

1. Begin by cook the beans.
2. Heat a drizzle of olive oil in a medium saucepan that has a lid over medium heat.
3. After the oil is warmed, add the onion let sauté for some minutes ensure to stir frequently till onions become translucent.
4. Add the chili cumin, powder, and cayenne blend.
5. Add the beans in ¼ cup of water stir to combine.
6. Cover the pan, reduce heat, let the beans cook by simmering for 10 minutes.
7. Remove from heat, mash some of the beans with the back of a big spoon.
8. Keep the pan until the meal is ready to serve.
9. Next, make the avocado salsa Verde by using a food processor.

10. In the food processor, combine the salsa Verde, cilantro, avocado, garlic clove, ½ of the jalapeño, and the juice of ½ lime.
11. Purée the salsa until it is super creamy.
12. Transfer the salsa Verde to a small saucepan and gently warm it over medium-low temperature as you stir frequently.
13. Cover the salsa and keep until you are ready to serve
14. Prepare the eggs and top with a light sprinkle of salt and pepper.
15. Warm the tortillas over low temperature gas.
16. Assemble the huevos rancheros by placing nn each plate, top tortilla with black beans, avocado sauce and egg.
17. Garnish with cilantro, chopped radishes, crumbled feta, and jalapeño.
18. Serve and enjoy with a bottle of hot sauce on the side.

Pumpkin pecan scones with maple glaze

Topped with a delightful maple glaze, this whole wheat pumpkin pecan makes a perfect healthy meal for your entire family in 30 minutes.

Ingredients

- ¾ cup of pumpkin puree
- ¼ cup of good maple syrup
- ½ teaspoon of vanilla extract
- 2 cups of white whole wheat flour
- ½ teaspoon of ginger
- ½ teaspoon of salt
- 1 cup of raw pecans
- ⅓ cup of solid coconut oil
- ¼ cup of milk of choice
- 1 teaspoon of cinnamon
- ¼ teaspoon of cloves or allspices
- 1 cup of powdered sugar
- 1 tablespoon of baking powder
- ¼ teaspoon of nutmeg
- ⅛ teaspoon of fine grain sea salt
- ¼ cup of brown sugar, packed
- 1 tablespoon of melted coconut oil or butter
- ½ teaspoon of vanilla

Directions

1. Preheat your oven to 425°F.
2. Place the nuts in a single layer on a rimmed baking sheet lined with parchment paper.
3. Toast the nuts in the oven for 3 minutes until fragrant.
4. Chop the nuts into fine pieces.
5. Combine the¾ of the chopped nuts, baking powder, flour, spices, sugar, and salt in a bowl then whisk at once.
6. Using a pastry cutter, cut the coconut oil into the dry ingredients.
7. Stir in pumpkin puree together with the milk and vanilla extract.
8. Mixing until you have thoroughly incorporated the wet and dry ingredients.
9. Form dough into a circle about an inch deep around.
10. Cut the circle into 8 even slices.
11. Separate slices and place on the baking sheet covered with parchment paper.
12. Bake for 15 – 17 minutes.
13. As the scones bake, whisk together the glaze ingredients in a small bowl until it forms a visible smooth and creamy.
14. Drizzle generously over the scones
15. While the glaze is wet, sprinkle it with the remaining chopped nuts.
16. Serve and enjoy.

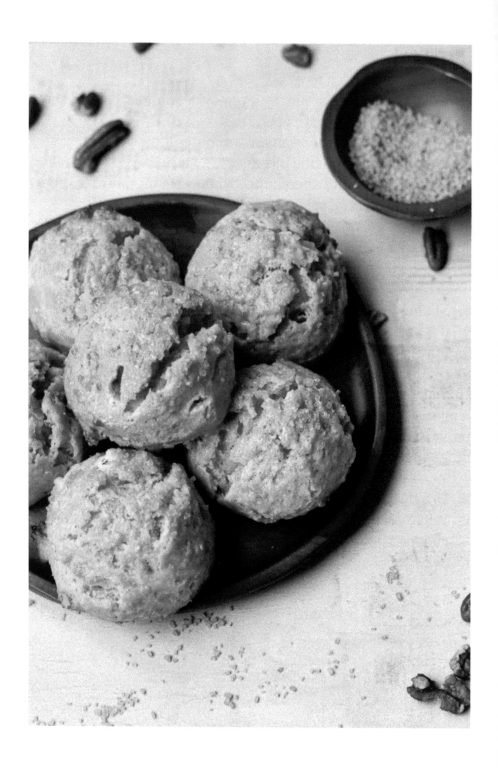